Unleashing the Secrets of the Mediterranean Diet!

"Revitalize Your Health and Unleash the Power of the Mediterranean Diet: Discover a World of Wellness Through Fresh Flavors and Lifelong Vitality!"

Angela MARSHALL

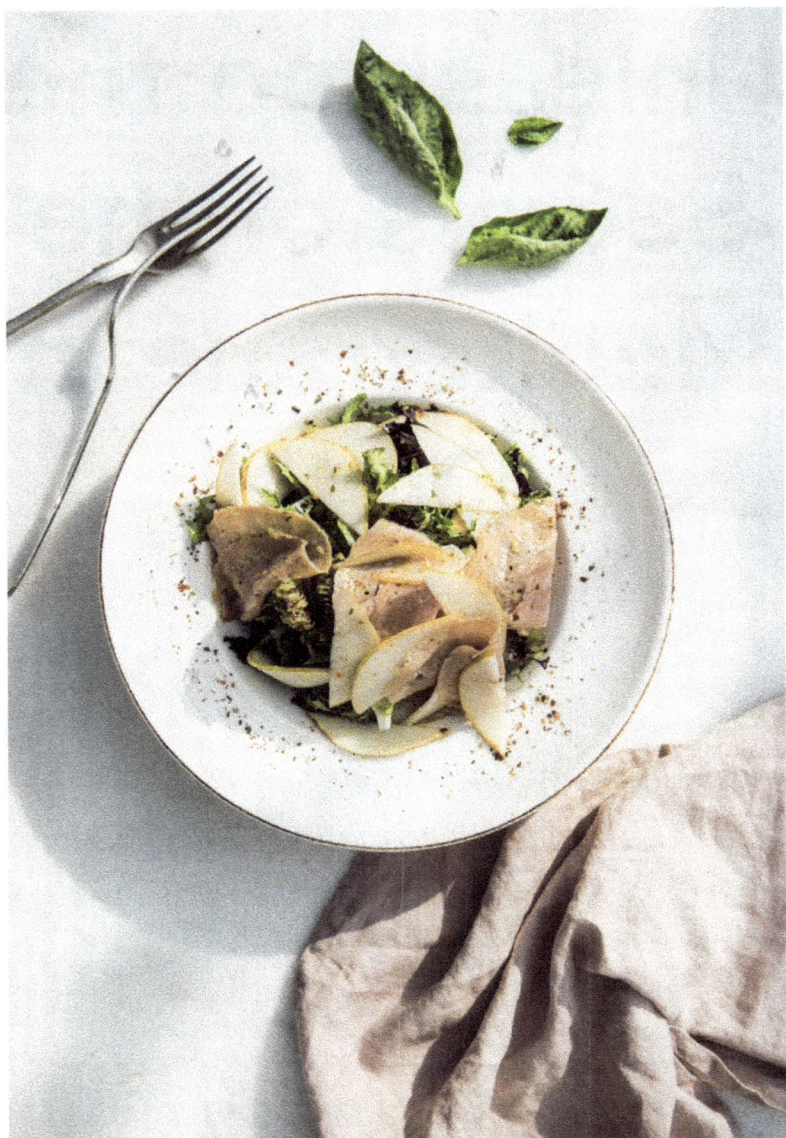

Table of content

MEDITERRANEAN BREAKFAST RECIPE

Greek Breakfast Pitas

Total time: 20 minutes

Prep time: 10 minutes

Cook time: 10 minutes

Yield: 4 servings

Ingredients

- ¼ cup chopped onion
- ¼ cup sweet red/black pepper, chopped
- 1 cup large egg
- ⅛ tsp. sea salt
- ⅛ tsp. black pepper
- 1 ½ tsp. fresh basil, ground
- ½ cup baby spinach, freshly torn
- 1 red tomato, sliced
- 2 pita bread, whole
- 2 tbsp. feta cheese, crumbled

Directions

- Coat a sizeable nonstick skillet with cooking spray and set over medium heat.
- Add onions and red peppers and sauté for at least 3 minutes.
- In a small bowl, beat together egg, pepper and salt and add the mixture to the skillet.
- Cook, stirring continuously, until ready.

- Spoon basil, spinach, and tomatoes onto the pitas and top with the egg mixture.
- Sprinkle with feta and serve.

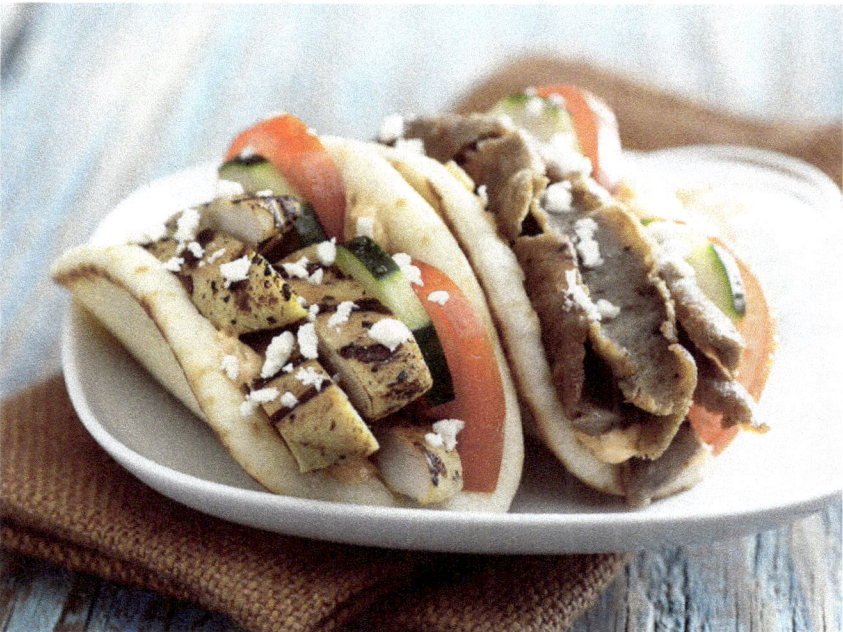

Healthy Breakfast Scramble

Total time: 20 minutes

Prep time: 5 minutes

Cook time: 15 minutes

Yield: 2 servings

Ingredients

- 1 tsp. extra virgin olive
- 4 medium green onions, chopped
- 1 tsp. dried basil leaves or 1 tbsp. fresh basil leaves, chopped
- 1 medium tomato, chopped
- 4 eggs
- Freshly ground pepper

Directions

- In a medium nonstick skillet, heat olive oil over medium heat; sauté green onions, stirring occasionally, for about 2 minutes.
- Stir in basil and tomato and let cook, stirring occasionally, for about 1 minute or until the tomato is cooked through.
- In a small bowl, thoroughly beat the eggs with a wire whisk or a fork and pour over the tomato mixture; cook for about 2 minutes.

- Gently lift the cooked parts with spatula to allow the uncooked parts to flow to the bottom.
- Continue cooking for about 3 minutes or until the eggs are cooked through.
- Season with pepper and serve.

Greek Parfait

Total time: 6 minutes

Prep time: 6 minutes

Cook time: 0 minutes

Yield: 6 servings

Ingredients

- 1 tsp. vanilla extract
- 3 cups low-fat Greek yogurt
- ¼ cup toasted unsalted pistachios, shelled
- 4 tsp. raw honey
- 28 Clementine segments

Directions

- In a mixing bowl, combine the vanilla extract with the Greek yogurt.
- Spoon ¼ cup of the mixture into 4 small parfait glasses.
- Top each of the 4 glasses with ½ tablespoon nuts, ½ teaspoon honey and 5 Clementine sections.
- Add the remaining yogurt mixture to the parfait glasses and top with ½ tablespoon nuts, Clementine segments and ½ teaspoon honey.
- Serve immediately

Quiche Wrapped in Prosciutto

Total time: 25 minutes

Prep time: 10 minutes

Cook time: 15 minutes

Yield: 8 servings

Ingredients

- 4 slices prosciutto, halved
- 2 egg whites
- 1 egg
- ½ tsp. rosemary, fresh and chopped and a little more for garnishing
- 3tbsp. low fat Greek yoghurt
- 1 tbsp. chopped black olives
- A pinch of black pepper, freshly ground   A pinch of salt

Directions

- Preheat your oven to 400°F and coat your muffin baking tray with cooking spray.
- Place each prosciutto piece into eight cups of the tray.
- In a medium bowl, whisk the egg whites and the egg until smooth.
- Pour in the yogurt, rosemary, olives, pepper, and salt and continue whisking.
- Divide the mixture equally among the prosciutto cups and bake uncovered until cooked through (about 15 minutes).
- Garnish with rosemary.

Morning Couscous

Total time: 35 minutes

Prep time 10 minutes

Cook time 25 minutes

Yield: 4 servings

Ingredients

- 3 cups soy milk
- 1 cinnamon stick
- 1 cup whole-wheat couscous, uncooked
- ¼ cup currants, dried
- ½ cup apricots, dried
- 4 tsp. sun butter, melted and divided
- 6 tsp. brown sugar, divided
- 1 pinch salt

Directions

- Put a saucepan on medium heat and pour in soy milk and the cinnamon stick.
- Let it heat for 3 minutes or until tiny bubbles start forming on the inner part of the pan; do not let it boil.
- Remove the saucepan from the heat and stir in the couscous, currants, apricots, salt, and 4 tablespoons of sugar.

- Put a lid on the pan and let it stand for 20 minutes. Remove the cinnamon stick.
- Divide the couscous among 4 bowls and top with ½ teaspoon of sugar and 1 teaspoon melted sun butter.
- Serve hot.

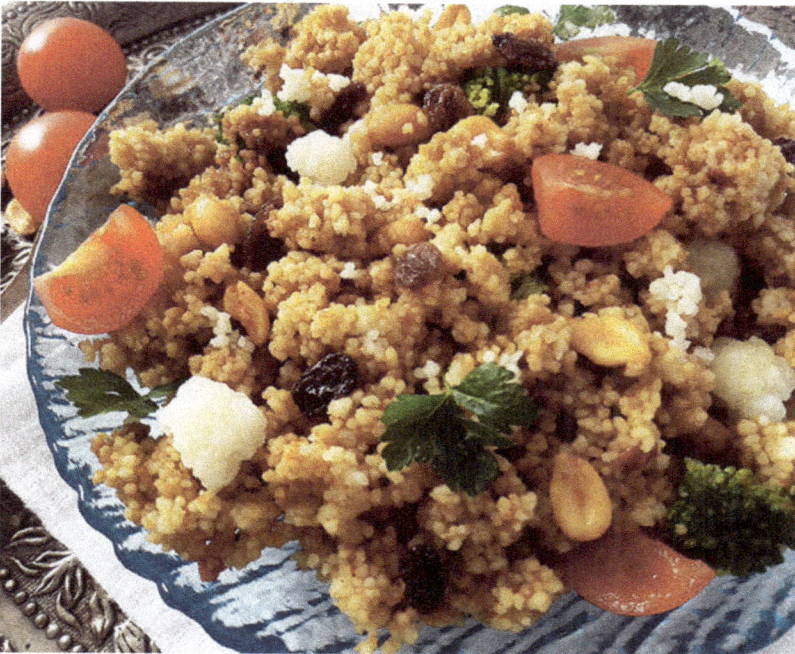

MEDITERRANEAN LUNCH RECIPE

Mediterranean Lettuce Wraps

Ingredients

- ¼ cup tahini
- ¼ cup extra-virgin olive oil
- 1 teaspoon lemon zest
- ¼ cup lemon juice (from 2 lemons)
- 1 ½ teaspoons pure maple syrup
- ¾ teaspoon kosher salt
- ½ teaspoon paprika
- 2 (15 ounce) cans no-salt-added chickpeas, rinsed
- ½ cup sliced jarred roasted red peppers, drained
- ½ cup thinly sliced shallots
- 12 large Bibb lettuce leaves
- ¼ cup toasted almonds, chopped
- 2 tablespoons chopped fresh parsley

Directions

- Whisk tahini, oil, lemon zest, lemon juice, maple syrup, salt and paprika in a large bowl. Add chickpeas, peppers and shallots. Toss to coat.
- Divide the mixture among lettuce leaves (about 1/3 cup each). Top with almonds and parsley. Wrap the lettuce leaves around the filling and serve.

Salmon Pita Sandwich

Ingredients

- 2 tablespoons plain nonfat yogurt
- 2 teaspoons chopped fresh dill
- 2 teaspoons lemon juice
- ½ teaspoon prepared horseradish
- 3 ounces flaked drained canned sockeye salmon
- ½ 6-inch whole-wheat pita bread
- ½ cup watercress

Directions

- Combine yogurt, dill, lemon juice and horseradish in a small bowl; stir in salmon. Stuff the pita half with the salmon salad and watercress.

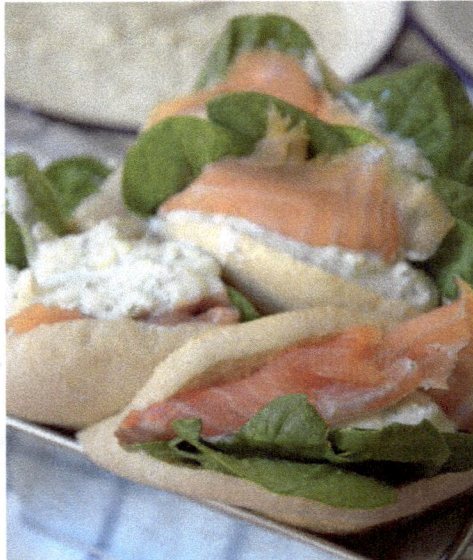

Hummus & Greek Salad

Ingredients

- 2 cups arugula
- ⅓ cup cherry tomatoes, halved
- ⅓ cup sliced cucumber
- 1 tablespoon chopped red onion
- 1 ½ tablespoons extra-virgin olive oil
- 2 teaspoons red-wine vinegar
- ⅛ teaspoon ground pepper
- 1 tablespoon feta cheese
- 1 4-inch whole-wheat pita
- ¼ cup hummus

Directions

- Toss arugula in a bowl with tomatoes, cucumber, onion, oil, vinegar and pepper. Top with feta. Serve with pita and hummus.

Mediterranean Wrap

Ingredients

- ½ cup water
- ⅓ cup couscous, preferably whole-wheat
- 1 cup chopped fresh parsley
- ½ cup chopped fresh mint
- ¼ cup lemon juice
- 3 tablespoons extra-virgin olive oil
- 2 teaspoons minced garlic
- ¼ teaspoon salt, divided
- ¼ teaspoon freshly ground pepper
- 1 pound chicken tenders
- 1 medium tomato, chopped
- 1 cup chopped cucumber
- 4 10-inch spinach or sun-dried tomato wraps or tortillas

Directions

- Bring water to a boil in a small saucepan. Stir in couscous and remove from the heat. Cover and let stand for 5 minutes. Fluff with a fork. Set aside.
- Meanwhile, combine parsley, mint, lemon juice, oil, garlic, 1/8 teaspoon salt and pepper in a small bowl.
- Toss chicken tenders in a medium bowl with 1 tablespoon of the parsley mixture and the remaining 1/8 teaspoon salt. Place the tenders in a large nonstick skillet and cook over medium heat until cooked though, 3 to 5 minutes per side.

Transfer to a clean cutting board. Cut into bite-size pieces when cool enough to handle.

- Stir the remaining parsley mixture into the couscous along with tomato and cucumber.

- To assemble wraps, spread about 3/4 cup of the couscous mixture onto each wrap. Divide the chicken among the wraps. Roll the wraps up like a burrito, tucking in the sides to hold the ingredients in. Serve cut in half.

Mediterranean Bento Lunch

Ingredients

- ¼ cup chickpeas, rinsed
- ¼ cup diced cucumber
- ¼ cup diced tomato
- 1 tablespoon diced olives
- 1 tablespoon crumbled feta cheese
- 1 tablespoon chopped fresh parsley
- ½ teaspoon extra-virgin olive oil
- 1 teaspoon red-wine vinegar
- 3 ounces grilled turkey breast tenderloin or chicken breast
- 1 cup grapes
- 1 whole-wheat pita bread, quartered
- 2 tablespoons hummus

Directions

- Toss chickpeas, cucumber, tomato, olives, feta, parsley, oil and vinegar together in a medium bowl. Pack in a medium-sized container.
- Place turkey (or chicken) in a medium container.
- Pack grapes and pita in small containers and hummus in a dip-size container.

Greek Chicken & Cucumber Pita Sandwiches with Yogurt Sauce

Ingredients

- 1 teaspoon lemon zest
- 2 tablespoons fresh lemon juice
- 5 teaspoons olive oil, divided
- 1 tablespoon chopped fresh oregano or 1 teaspoon dried
- 2 ¾ teaspoons minced garlic, divided
- ¼ teaspoon crushed red pepper
- 1 pound chicken tenders
- 1 English cucumber, halved, seeded and grated, plus 1/2 English cucumber, halved and sliced
- ½ teaspoon salt, divided
- ¾ cup nonfat plain Greek yogurt
- 2 teaspoons chopped fresh mint
- 2 teaspoons chopped fresh dill
- 1 teaspoon ground pepper
- 2 (6 1/2 inch) whole-wheat pita breads, halved
- 4 lettuce leaves
- ½ cup sliced red onion
- 1 cup chopped plum tomatoes

Directions

- Combine lemon zest, lemon juice, 3 tsp. oil, oregano, 2 tsp. garlic, and crushed red pepper in a large bowl. Add chicken and toss to coat. Marinate in the refrigerator for at least 1 hour or up to 4 hours.

- Meanwhile, toss grated cucumber with 1/4 tsp. salt in a fine-mesh sieve. Let drain for 15 minutes, then squeeze to release more liquid. Transfer to a medium bowl. Stir in yogurt, mint, dill, ground pepper, and the remaining 2 tsp. oil, 3/4 tsp. garlic, and 1/4 tsp. salt. Refrigerate until ready to serve.

- Preheat grill to medium-high.

- Oil the grill rack (see Tip). Grill the chicken until an instant-read thermometer inserted in the center registers 165 degrees F, 3 to 4 minutes per side.

- To serve, spread some of the sauce inside each pita half. Tuck in the chicken, lettuce, red onion, tomatoes, and sliced cucumber.

Slow-Cooker Mediterranean Chicken & Chickpea Soup

Ingredients

- 1 ½ cups dried chickpeas, soaked overnight
- 4 cups water
- 1 large yellow onion, finely chopped
- 1 (15 ounce) can no-salt-added diced tomatoes, preferably fire-roasted
- 2 tablespoons tomato paste
- 4 cloves garlic, finely chopped
- 1 bay leaf
- 4 teaspoons ground cumin
- 4 teaspoons paprika
- ¼ teaspoon cayenne pepper
- ¼ teaspoon ground pepper
- 2 pounds bone-in chicken thighs, skin removed, trimmed
- 1 (14 ounce) can artichoke hearts, drained and quartered
- ¼ cup halved pitted oil-cured olives
- ½ teaspoon salt
- ¼ cup chopped fresh parsley or cilantro

Directions

- Drain chickpeas and place in a 6-quart or larger slow cooker. Add 4 cups water, onion, tomatoes and their juice, tomato paste, garlic, bay leaf, cumin, paprika, cayenne and ground pepper; stir to combine. Add chicken.
- Cover and cook on Low for 8 hours or High for 4 hours.

- Transfer the chicken to a clean cutting board and let cool slightly. Discard bay leaf. Add artichokes, olives and salt to the slow cooker and stir to combine. Shred the chicken, discarding bones. Stir the chicken into the soup. Serve topped with parsley (or cilantro).

MEDITERRANEAN SALAD RECIPES

Potato Salad

Total time: 24 minutes

Prep time: 10 minutes

Cook time: 14 minutes

Yield: 4 servings

Ingredients

- 5 medium potatoes, peeled and diced
- Coarse salt, to taste
- ¼ onion
- 3 tbsp. yellow mustard
- 2 cups mayonnaise
- 1 tsp. paprika, sweet
- 1 tsp. Tabasco
- 2 scallions, thinly sliced

Directions

- Pour some water in a saucepan and place over medium heat.
- Add the potatoes, season with coarse salt and boil for around 10 minutes until tender.
- Drain the water and return the saucepan to the heat to dry them out.
- Let the potatoes cool to room temperature.
- Grate the onion in a mixing bowl, add mustard, mayo, paprika and the hot sauce and mix well.
- Add the potatoes to the bowl and toss until evenly coated.
- Divide among four bowls and top with the sliced scallions.

Mediterranean Green Salad

Total time: 25 minutes

Prep time: 15 minutes

Cook time: 10 minutes

Yield: 4 servings

Ingredients

- ½ loaf rustic sourdough bread
- ¼ tsp. paprika
- 2 tbsp. manchego, finely grated
- 7 tbsp. extra virgin olive oil, divided
- 1 ½ tbsp. sherry vinegar
- ½ tsp. sea salt
- 1 tsp. freshly ground black pepper
- 1 tsp. Dijon mustard
- 5 cups mixed baby greens
- ¾ cup green olives, pitted and halved
- 12 thin slices of Serrano ham, roughly chopped

Directions

- Cut the bread into bite-sized cubes and set aside.
- Preheat oven to 400°F.
- In a mixing bowl, combine paprika, manchego and 6 tbsps. of olive oil.
- Add the bread cubes and toss them until they are evenly coated with the flavored oil.
- Arrange the bread on a baking sheet and bake for about 8 minutes until golden brown and let the bread cool.

- In a separate bowl, combine the vinegar, salt, pepper, mustard and the remaining olive oil.
- Add this mixture to a larger bowl containing the greens until they are lightly coated with the vinaigrette.
- Add all the other ingredients and the croutons and toss well.
- Serve the salad on four plates.

Chickpea Salad with Yogurt Dressing

Total time: 30 minutes

Prep time: 30 minutes

Cook time: 0 minutes

Yield: 4 servings

Ingredients

Dressing

- 1 tbsp. freshly squeezed lemon juice
- 1 cup plain nonfat Greek yogurt
- ¼ tsp. cayenne pepper
- 1½ tsp. curry powder

Salad

- 2 15-oz. cans chickpeas, rinsed and drained
- 1 cup diced red apple
- ½ cup diced celery
- ¼ cup chopped walnuts
- ¼ cup thinly sliced green onions
- ⅓ cup raisins
- ½ cup chopped fresh parsley
- 2 lemon wedges

Directions

- Make dressing: In a small bowl, whisk together lemon juice, yogurt, cayenne, and curry powder until well combined.
- Make salad: In a large bowl, toss together chickpeas, apple, celery, walnuts, green onions, raisins, and parsley.
- Gently fold in the dressing and season with sea salt and pepper.
- Serve garnished with lemon wedges.

MEDITERRANEAN POULTRY RECIPES

Grilled Turkey with Salsa

Total time: 50 minutes

Prep time: 15 minutes

Cook time: 35 minutes

Yield: 6 servings

Ingredients

For the spice rub:

- 1 ½ tsp. garlic powder
- 1 ½ tsp. sweet paprika
- 2 tsp. crushed fennel seeds
- 2 tsp. dark brown sugar
- 1 tsp. sea salt
- 1 ½ tsp. freshly ground black pepper

For the salsa:

- 2 tbsp. drained capers
- ¼ cup pimento-stuffed green olives, chopped
- 2 scant cups cherry tomatoes, diced
- 1 ½ tbsp. extra virgin olive oil
- 1 large clove garlic, minced
- 2 tbsp. torn fresh basil leaves
- 2 tsp. fresh lemon juice
- ½ tsp. finely grated lemon zest
- 6 turkey breast cutlets
- 1 cup diced red onion
- Sea salt
- Freshly ground black pepper

Directions

- Mix together garlic powder, paprika, fennel seeds, brown sugar, salt and pepper in a small bowl.
- In another bowl, combine capers, olives, tomatoes, onion extra virgin olive oil, garlic, basil, lemon juice and zest, ¼ teaspoon sea salt and pepper; set aside.
- Grill the meat on medium high heat after dipping in the spice rub for about 3 minutes per side or until browned on both sides.
- Transfer the grilled turkey to a serving plate and let rest for about 5 minutes.
- Serve with salsa.

Curried Chicken with Olives, Apricots and Cauliflower

Total time: 8 hours 50 minutes

Refrigerator time: 8 hours

Prep time: 15 minutes

Cook time: 35 minutes

Yield: 4 to 6 servings

Ingredients

- 8 chicken thighs, skinless, boneless
- ¼ cup extra virgin olive oil, divided
- ½ tsp. ground cinnamon
- ¼ tsp. cayenne pepper
- 1 tsp. smoked paprika, divided
- 4 tsp. curry powder, divided
- 1 tbsp. apple cider vinegar
- Sea salt, to taste
- 1 head cauliflower, chopped
- 1 cup pitted green olives, halved
- ¾ cup dried apricots, chopped, soaked in hot water and drained
- ⅓ cup chopped fresh cilantro
- 6 lemon wedges

Directions

- Combine chicken thighs, 2 tablespoons extra virgin olive oil, cinnamon, cayenne, ½ teaspoon paprika, 2 tablespoons curry powder, vinegar, and sea salt in a medium bowl; toss to coat and refrigerate covered, for about 8 hours.
- Position rack in the center of oven and preheat oven to 450ºF.
- Prepare a rimmed sheet pan by lining it with parchment paper; add cauliflower and remaining olive oil, paprika, and curry powder; mix well.
- Add olives and apricots and spread the mixture in a single layer.
- Place the marinated chicken on top of the cauliflower mixture, spacing evenly apart, and roast in the preheated oven for about 35 minutes or until chicken is cooked through and cauliflower browns.
- Serve the cauliflower and chicken sprinkled with cilantro and garnished with lemon wedges.

Chicken Salad with Pine Nuts, Raisins and Fennel

Total time: 10 minutes

Prep time: 10 minutes

Cook time: 0 minutes

Chill time: 1 hour

Yield: 1 large bowl

Ingredients

For the dressing:

- 1 tbsp. extra virgin olive oil
- 3 tbsp. mayonnaise
- ½ small clove garlic, mashed with sea salt
- Pinch cayenne
- 1 tbsp. freshly squeezed fresh lemon juice

For the salad:

- 3 tbsp. chopped sweet onion
- ⅓ cup small-diced fresh fennel
- 1 cup shredded cooked chicken
- 2 tbsp. golden raisins
- 2 tbsp. toasted pine nuts
- 2 tbsp. chopped fresh flat-leaf parsley
- Sea salt
- Freshly ground pepper

Directions

- Combine extra virgin olive oil, mayonnaise, garlic, cayenne, and lemon juice in a small bowl; mix well.
- In a separate bowl, mix onion, fennel, chicken, raisins, pine nuts, and parsley; gently add in the dressing and fold the ingredients together. Season with sea salt and pepper and refrigerate for at least 1 hour for flavors to meld before serving.

Slow Cooker Rosemary Chicken

Total time: 7 hours 20 minutes

Prep time: 20 minutes

Cook time: 7 hours, 10 minutes

Yield: 8 servings

Ingredients

- 1 small onion, thinly sliced
- 4 cloves garlic, pressed
- 1 medium red bell pepper, sliced
- 2 tsp. dried rosemary
- ½ tsp. dried oregano
- 2 pork sausages
- 8 chicken breasts, skinned, deboned and halved
- ¼ tsp. coarsely ground pepper
- ¼ cup dry vermouth
- 1 ½ tbsp. corn starch
- 2 tbsp. cold water

Directions

- Combine onion, garlic, bell pepper, rosemary and oregano in a slow cooker.
- Crumble the sausages over the mixture, casings removed.
- Arrange the chicken in a single layer over the sausage and sprinkle with pepper.
- Add the vermouth and slow-cook for 7 hours.

- Warm a deep platter, move the chicken to the platter and cover.
- Mix the cornstarch with the water in a small bowl and add this to the liquid in the slow cooker.
- Increase the heat and cover.
- Cook for about 10 minutes.

MEDITERRANEAN SEAFOOD RECIPES

Fish with Olives, Tomatoes, and Capers

Total time: 21 minutes

Prep time: 5 minutes

Cook time: 16 minutes

Yield: 4 servings

Ingredients

- 4 tsp. extra virgin olive oil, divided
- 4 (5-ounce) sea bass fillets
- 1 small onion, diced
- ½ cup white wine
- 2 tbsp. capers
- 1 cup canned diced tomatoes, with juice
- ½ cup pitted black olives, chopped
- ¼ tsp. crushed red pepper
- 2 cups fresh baby spinach leaves
- Sea salt and pepper

Directions

- Heat 2 teaspoons of extra virgin olive oil in a large nonstick skillet set over medium high heat.
- Add fish and cook for about 3 minutes per side or until opaque in the center.
- Transfer the cooked fish to a plate and keep warm.
- Add the remaining oil to the skillet and sauté onion for about 2 minutes or until translucent.
- Stir in wine and cook for about 2 minutes or until liquid is reduced by half.

- Stir in capers, tomatoes, olives, and red pepper and cook for about 3 minutes more.
- Add spinach and cook, stirring for about 3 minutes or until silted.
- Stir in sea salt and pepper and spoon sauce over fish.
- Serve immediately.

Mediterranean Cod

Total time: 50 minutes

Prep time: 15 minutes

Cook time: 35 minutes

Yield: 4 servings

Ingredients

- 1 tbsp. extra virgin olive oil
- 100g frozen chopped onion
- 1 tbsp. frozen chopped garlic
- 230g can Italian tomatoes, chopped
- 1 tbsp. tomato purée
- 400g pack skinless and boneless cod fillets
- 200g frozen mixed peppers
- 1 tbsp. chopped frozen parsley
- 50g pitted black olives
- 800g package frozen white rice

Directions

- Add extra virgin olive oil to a saucepan set over medium heat; stir in onion and sauté for about 3 minutes.
- Add garlic and sauté for 2 minutes more or until fragrant.
- Stir in the tomatoes, tomato puree, and water and bring to a gentle boil.
- Reduce heat and simmer for about 20 minutes or until thickened.

- Add cod and peppers; nudge the fish in the sauce a bit and bring back to a boil; lower heat and simmer for about 8 minutes.
- Sprinkle with parsley and olives and simmer for 2 minutes more.
- In the meantime, follow package instructions to cook rice.
- Serve fish with hot rice.

BIANKO FROM CORFU

Serves 4

- 1⁄2 cup extra-virgin olive oil, divided 2 large onions, peeled and sliced
- 6 cloves garlic, peeled and minced
- 2 medium carrots, peeled and sliced
- 1 cup chopped celery
- 1 1⁄2 teaspoons salt, divided 1 teaspoon pepper, divided
- 4 large potatoes, peeled and cut into 1⁄2-inch slices
- 4 whitefish fillets (cod or grouper), skinned
- 3–5 tablespoons fresh lemon juice
- 1⁄4 cup chopped fresh parsley

Directions

- Heat 1⁄4 cup of oil in a heavy-bottomed pot over medium heat for 30 seconds. Add the onions, garlic, carrots, and celery. Cook the vegetables for 5–7 minutes or until the onions soften. Then season them with 1⁄2 teaspoon of salt and 1⁄4 teaspoon of pepper.
- Add the potatoes and the remaining salt and pepper. Add just enough hot water to cover the potatoes. Increase the heat to medium-high and bring the water to a boil. Reduce the heat to medium-low, cover the pot, leaving the lid slightly ajar, and cook for 12 minutes.
- Place the fillets over the potatoes and top with the remaining oil. Cover the fish and cook for another 12–15 minutes or until the whitefish is opaque and flaky.

- Uncover the pot and add the lemon juice. Don't stir it; shake the pot back and forth to allow the juice to penetrate the layers. Adjust the seasoning with more salt and pepper, if necessary.
- Place the fish and potatoes on a large platter and top with the parsley. Serve immediately.

GRILLED SALMON WITH LEMON AND LIME

Serves 4

- 4 (6-ounce) salmon fillets, skins on
- 1⁄4 cup extra-virgin olive oil
- 1 tablespoon grated lemon zest
- 11⁄2 teaspoons grated lime zest
- 11⁄2 teaspoons salt
- 1⁄2 teaspoon pepper
- 3 tablespoons vegetable oil
- 1 large lemon, cut into wedges

Directions

- Preheat a gas or charcoal grill to medium-high. Brush the grill surface to make sure it is thoroughly clean. Rinse the fillets and pat them dry with a paper towel. Rub the fillets with the olive oil on both sides.
- Sprinkle both sides of the fillets with the lemon zest, lime zest, salt, and pepper.
- When the grill is ready, dip a clean tea towel in the vegetable oil and wipe the grill surface with the oil.
- Place the salmon on the grill, skin-side down, and grill for 6–7 minutes. Don't touch the fillets, just let them grill. Flip the salmon over and grill for another 2–3 minutes.
- Serve the salmon with lemon wedges.

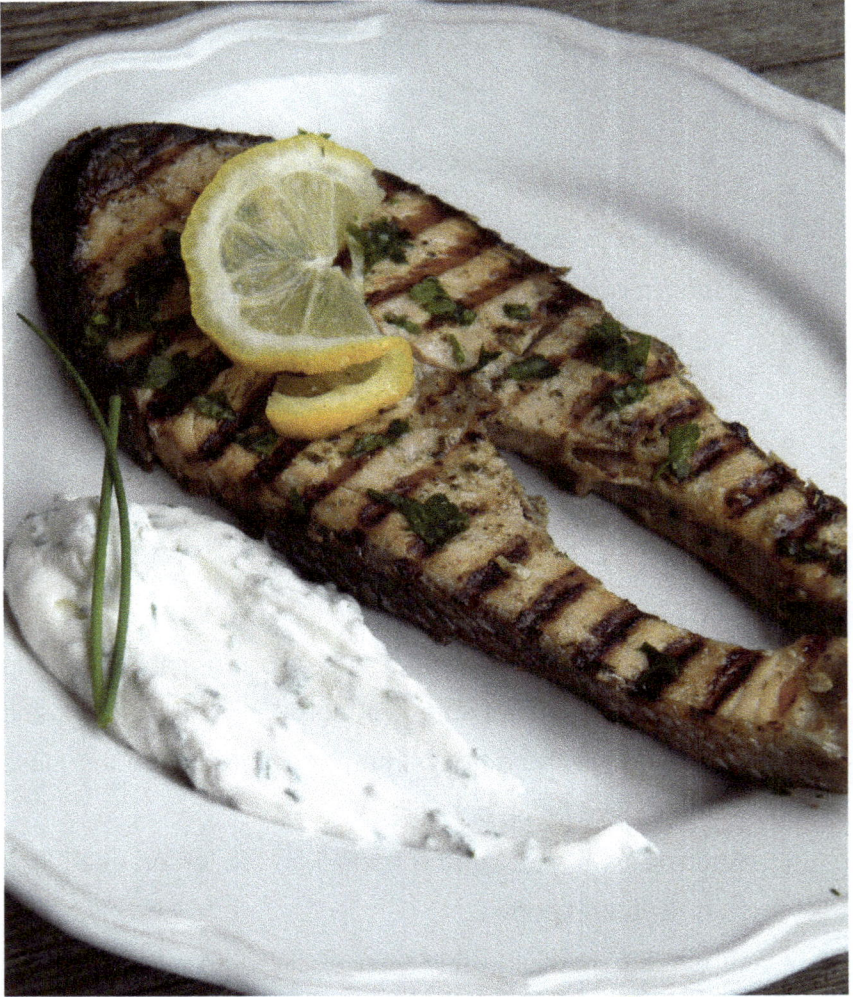

MEDITERRANEAN MEAT, BEEF AND PORK RECIPES

Roasted Pork With Balsamic Sauce

Total time: 1 hour

Prep time: 20 minutes

Cook time: 40 minutes

Yield: 6 servings

Ingredients

- 1 tsp. extra virgin olive oil
- 1 clove garlic, minced
- ¼ cup diced yellow onion
- 1 ½ cups low-sodium vegetable or chicken broth
- ¼ cup balsamic vinegar
- ½ cup port
- ¼ cup dried cherries
- ½ cup 2% milk
- ¼ cup low-fat sour cream
- ¾ lb. pork tenderloin, trimmed

Directions

- Heat extra virgin olive oil in a medium saucepan set over medium high heat; add garlic and onion and sauté for about 3 minutes or until tender.
- Stir in chicken broth, balsamic vinegar, port, and dried cherries and cook until the sauce is reduced to ½ cup.

- Scrape the sauce into the blender and blend until very smooth; stir in milk and sour cream and return to pan; stir until heated through.
- Preheat your oven to 375°F.
- Place pork tenderloin into a roasting pan and roast in the oven for about 15 minutes.
- Remove pork from oven and let rest for about 5 minutes and then slice into small slices. Serve the meat over 3 tablespoons of sauce.

Mediterranean Beef Pitas

Total time: 15 minutes

Prep time: 10 minutes

Cook time: 5 minutes

Yield: 4 servings

Ingredients

- 1pound ground beef
- Freshly ground black pepper
- Sea salt
- 1 ½ tsp. dried oregano
- 2 tbsp. extra virgin olive oil, divided
- ¼ small red onion, sliced
- 3/4cup store-bought hummus
- 2 tbsp. fresh flat-leaf parsley
- 4 pitas
- 4 lemon wedges

Directions

- Form beef into 16 patties; season with ¼ teaspoon ground pepper, ½ teaspoon sea salt and oregano.
- Add 1 tablespoon of extra virgin olive oil in a skillet set over medium heat; cook the beef patties for about 2 minutes per side or until lightly browned. To serve, top pitas with the beef patties, hummus, parsley and onion and drizzle with the remaining extra virgin olive oil; garnish with lemon wedges.

Parmesan Meat Loaf

Total time: 1 hour

Prep time: 10 minutes

Cook time: 50 minutes

Yield: 4 servings

Ingredients

- 1½ pounds ground beef
- ½ cup bread crumbs
- ½ cup chopped flat-leaf parsley
- 1 grated onion
- 1 large egg
- ½ cup grated Parmesan
- ¼ cup tomato paste
- Sea salt
- Freshly ground black pepper

Directions

- Preheat your oven to 400ºF. In a large bowl, mix together ground beef, bread crumbs, parsley, onion, egg, Parmesan cheese, tomato paste, sea salt and pepper.
- Line a baking sheet with foil and add the beef mixture, pressing to form an 8-inch loaf.
- Bake in the preheated oven for about 50 minutes or until cooked through.

Mediterranean Flank Steak

Total time: 1 hour

Prep time: 20 minutes

Cook time: 40 minutes

Yield: 4 to 6 servings

Ingredients

- 2 tbsp. chopped aromatic herbs (marjoram, rosemary, sage, thyme, or a mix)
- 2 cloves garlic, minced
- 2 tbsp. extra virgin olive oil
- 1 tbsp. sea salt
- 1 tbsp. ground black pepper
- 1½-to 2-lb. flank steak, trimmed
- ½ cup Greek vinaigrette

Directions

- In a small bowl, mix together herbs, garlic, extra virgin olive oil, sea salt, and pepper; rub over the steak and let rest for about 20 minutes.
- In the meantime, heat your gas grill to medium high.
- Grill the steak for about 15 minutes, turning meat every 4 minutes for even cooking.
- Transfer the cooked steak to a cutting board and let rest for about 5 minutes; slice into small slices and place on plates.
- Drizzle with vinaigrette and serve immediately.

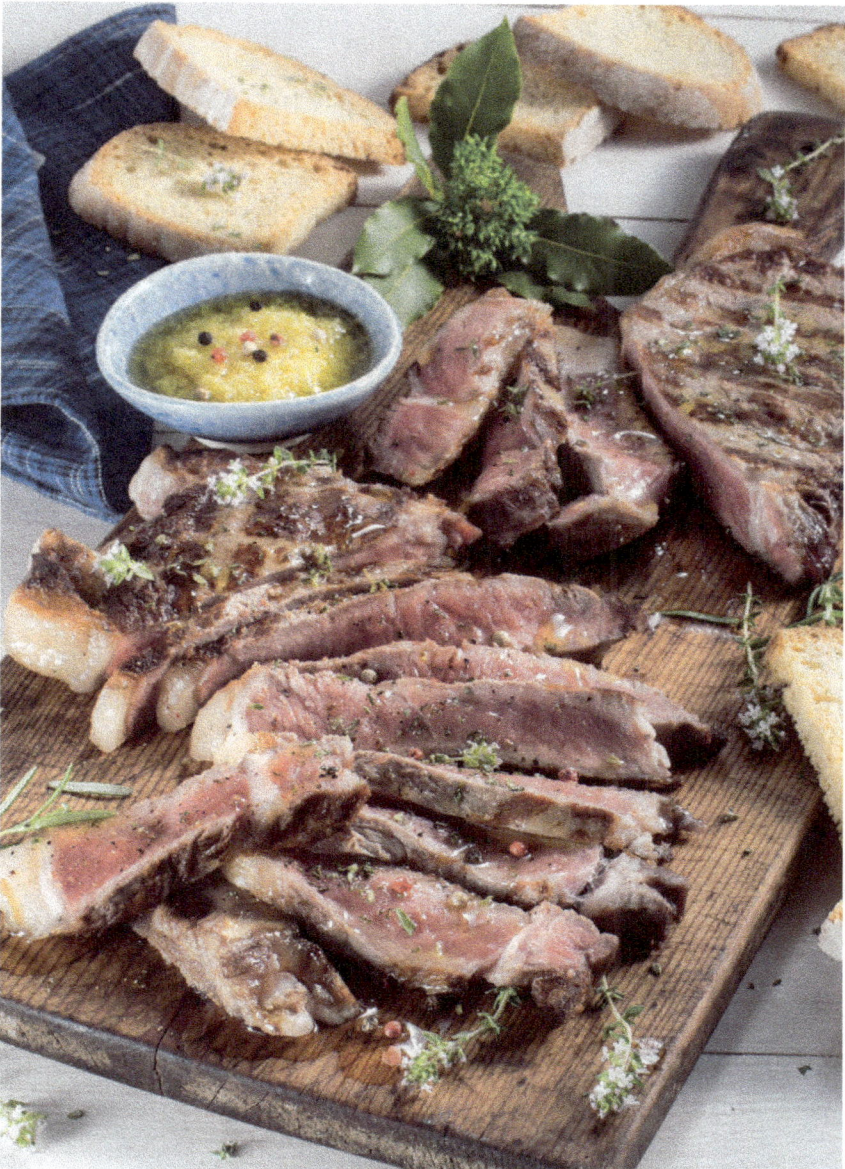

VEGETARIAN AND LEGUMES MEDITERRANEAN RECIPES

Green Bean and Zucchini Sauté

Total time: 15 minutes

Prep time: 5 minutes

Cook time: 10 minutes

Yield: 4 servings

Ingredients

- 7.5ml olive oil, divided
- 50g trimmed green beans - cut into small pieces
- ½ small zucchini, thinly sliced
- 2g red chili flakes
- 7.5ml lemon juice
- 15g sliced scallions
- 1g red chili flakes
- Handful of parmesan flakes
- 1g pepper
- 1g salt

Directions

- Add half of the oil to a skillet set over medium heat.
- Stir in green beans, zucchini, salt and pepper and sauté, stirring, for about 9 minutes or until the vegetables are crisp tender.
- Remove the pan from heat and stir in lemon juice, scallions.
- Serve garnished with red chili flakes and cheese.

Stuffed Grape Leaves Dish

Total time: 2 hours

Prep time: 30 minutes

Cook time: 1 hour 30 minutes

Yield: 8 servings

Ingredients

- 30 fresh grape leaves
- 2 tbsp. extra virgin olive oil
- 2 cups finely diced onion
- 1 cup brown rice
- 1 cup dried currants or raisins
- 1 cup chopped fresh mint
- 1 cup chopped fresh parsley
- 1 cup chopped hulled pistachios
- 2 cups tomato juice
- Sea salt and pepper, to taste
- Pomegranate molasses, to drizzle
- ¼ cup freshly squeezed lemon juice
- 1 lemon, sliced
- 1 tsp. extra virgin olive oil for brushing casserole dish and top of casserole

Directions

- Place grape leaves in a pot of boiling water; cook for about 2 minutes and remove from heat; drain, and set aside.

- In a large saucepan set over medium heat, heat extra virgin olive oil; add onion, and sauté for about 10 minutes or until lightly browned.
- Stir in rice and 2 ½ cups of water; bring to a gentle boil, cover and reduce heat to medium low.
- Cook for about 40 minutes or until rice is cooked through and water is absorbed.
- Remove the cooked rice from heat and stir in lemon juice, raisins, mint, parsley, pistachios, tomato juice, sea salt, and pepper.
- Preheat your oven to 350°F.
- Grease a 2-quart baking dish with extra virgin olive oil and line its bottom with grape leaves, allowing them to hang over the sides.
- With paper towels, pat the leaves dry and spread with half of the rice mixture.
- Top the rice mixture with more grape leaves and top with the remaining rice.
- Cover with the remaining leaves and fold over the leaves around edges to seal.
- Brush the top with extra virgin olive oil and bake in the preheated oven for about 40 minutes or until casserole is firm and dry and the grape leaves darken.
- Using a wet knife, cut the casserole into eight pieces and place each on eight plates.
- Drizzle each serving with pomegranate molasses and garnish with lemon slices.

Olive, Bell Pepper and Arugula Salsa

Total time: 30 minutes

Prep time: 25 minutes

Cook time: 5 minutes

Yield: 1 ½ cups

Ingredients

- 1 ½ tbsp. extra virgin olive oil
- 1 tsp. crushed fennel seeds
- 1 red and 1 yellow bell peppers, diced
- 16 pitted Kalamata olives, chopped
- Sea salt and pepper, to taste
- ½ cup chopped baby arugula

Directions

- In a large nonstick skillet, heat extra virgin olive oil; sauté fennel seeds for about 1 minute, stirring.
- Stir in bell peppers and continue sautéing for 4 minutes more or until peppers are tender.
- Scrape the pepper mixture into a bowl; stir in olives, sea salt, and pepper.
- Let stand for at least 2 minutes, stirring occasionally, for flavors to meld.
- Add in arugula, toss until slightly wilted, and serve.

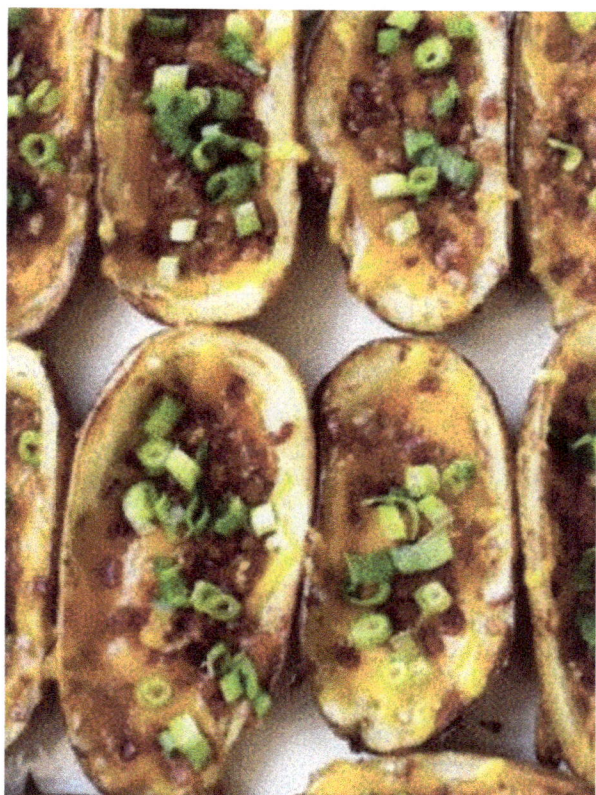

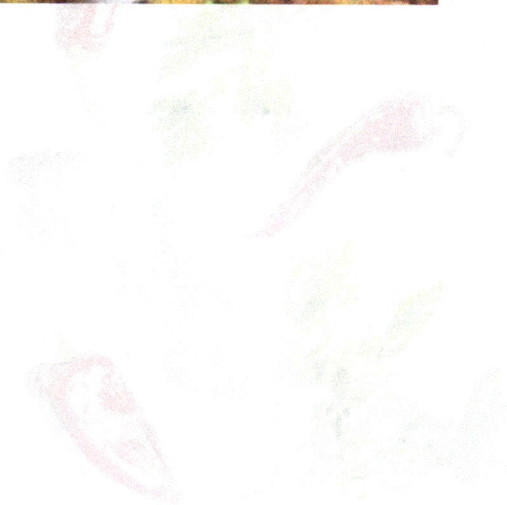

Roasted Pepper and Bean Dip

Total time: 10 minutes

Prep time: 10 minutes

Cook time: 0 minutes

Yield: 2 ½ Cups

Ingredients

- 1 (7-oz.) jar roasted red bell peppers
- 1 tbsp. extra virgin olive oil
- 1 16-oz. can cannellini beans, rinsed, drained
- 1 cup (6 oz.) light firm silken tofu
- 1 clove garlic, chopped
- ½ tsp. ground cumin
- 2 tbsp. freshly squeezed lime juice
- ⅓ cup cilantro leaves
- ½ tsp. sea salt

Directions

- Set aside ¼ cup of roasted peppers.
- Place the remaining roasted peppers in a food processor along with other ingredients; process until very smooth.
- Spoon the pepper mixture into a serving bowl; stir the reserved peppers into the mixture. Serve at room temperature or chilled.

MEDITERRANEAN DESSERTS

REVANI SYRUP CAKE

Serves 24

- 1 tablespoon unsalted butter
- 2 tablespoons all-purpose flour
- 1 cup ground rusk or bread crumbs
- 1 cup fine semolina flour
- 3/4 cup ground toasted almonds
- 3 teaspoons baking powder
- 16 large eggs
- 2 tablespoons vanilla extract
- 3 cups sugar, divided
- 3 cups water
- 5 (2-inch) strips lemon peel, pith removed
- 3 tablespoons fresh lemon juice
- 1 ounce brandy

Directions

- Preheat the oven to 350°F. Grease a 13" × 9" baking pan with the butter and then coat it with the flour.
- In a medium bowl, combine the rusk, semolina flour, almonds, and baking powder. In another medium bowl, whisk the eggs, vanilla, and 1 cup of sugar using an electric mixer on medium for 5 minutes or until the eggs turn a light yellow. Stir the semolina mixture into the eggs in three batches.
- Pour the batter into the baking pan, and bake it on the middle rack for 30–35 minutes or until a toothpick inserted

into the middle of the cake comes out clean. While the cake is baking, make the syrup. Bring the remaining sugar, water, and lemon peel to a boil in a medium pot over medium-high heat. Reduce the heat to medium-low and cook for 6 minutes. Add the lemon juice and cook for 3 minutes. Take the syrup off the heat and add the brandy. Let the syrup cool. Remove the lemon peel and reserve the syrup.

- When the cake is finished, ladle the syrup over it and let the cake soak up the syrup.
- Cut the cake into squares or diamond shapes. Serve the cake at room temperature; you can store leftovers in the refrigerator for up to one week.

CINNAMON ROLLS WITH TAHINI AND HONEY

Serves 16

- 1 cup whole milk, warm
- 2¼ teaspoons active dry yeast
- 3 tablespoons vegetable oil
- 3¼ cups unbleached all-purpose flour, divided
- ½ cup sugar 1 large egg
- 1 teaspoon salt
- ¾ cup (packed) golden brown sugar
- 2 tablespoons ground cinnamon
- ¾ cup tahini
- ¾ cup honey 1 teaspoon lemon zest
- 2 tablespoons lemon juice
- ¼ cup plus 1 tablespoon unsalted butter, at room temperature, divided

Directions

- In a large bowl, combine the warm milk and yeast. Set the mixture aside for 7–10 minutes to allow the yeast to activate. Stir in the oil, 1 cup of flour, sugar, egg, and salt. Using your hands, mix in 2 cups flour to form a soft dough that is not too sticky. Cover the dough with plastic wrap and let it rise for 2 hours or until it doubles in size.
- In a small bowl, thoroughly combine the brown sugar and cinnamon, and reserve it. In another small bowl, combine

the tahini, honey, lemon zest, and lemon juice. Stir to thoroughly combine and reserve.

- Grease a 13" × 9" baking pan with 1 tablespoon of butter. Spread the remaining flour on the work surface. After the dough rises, punch it down with your fist and place it on the floured surface. Roll the dough to a 9" × 14" rectangle. Spread the remaining butter over the surface of the dough, leaving a 1/2-inch border around the dough. Sprinkle the brown sugar mixture over the butter.

- Beginning at the longest end of the dough, roll the dough to form a tight cylinder. Cut the dough into sixteen equal slices. Place the slices in the pan leaving some space between them to allow them to rise. Cover the rolls with a tea towel and let them rise in a warm place for 3 hours or until they fill the pan. Preheat the oven to 375°F.

- Bake the rolls on the middle rack for 20–25 minutes or until they turn golden. Let the rolls cool for 5 minutes, and then smear the tahini topping over each one. Pull the rolls apart, and serve them warm or at room temperature.

PEAR CROUSTADE

Serves 8

- 1 cup plus 1 tablespoon all-purpose flour, divided
- 4 1/2 tablespoons sugar, divided 1/8 teaspoon salt 6 tablespoons unsalted butter, chilled, cut into 1/2-inch cubes 1 large egg, separated
- 1 1/2 tablespoons ice-cold water 3 firm ripe pears (Bosc), peeled, cored, sliced into 1/4-inch slices 1 tablespoon fresh lemon juice
- 1/3 teaspoon ground allspice 1 teaspoon anise seeds

Directions

- Put 1 cup flour, 1 1/2 tablespoons sugar, and salt into a food processor, and pulse to combine the ingredients. Add the butter and pulse until the mixture resembles coarse crumbs. Transfer the ingredients to a bowl.
- In another small bowl, whisk the egg yolk and ice water. Add the egg mixture to the flour-butter mixture, and stir to combine. Form a dough ball, and then flatten it into a disc. Wrap the dough in plastic wrap, and chill it for an hour.
- Preheat the oven to 400°F. Place the dough on parchment paper and roll it until it is 10 inches around. Transfer the dough and the parchment to a baking sheet.
- In a large bowl, add the pears, remaining sugar, remaining flour, lemon juice, allspice, and anise, and toss to combine the ingredients.

- Place the filling in the center of the dough and spread it out evenly, leaving a 2-inch border around the edges. Fold the dough border over the fruit to form a rustic edge. Pinch any dough that has cracked to seal it. In a small bowl, whisk the egg white and brush it over the dough.
- Place the baking sheet on the middle rack of the oven, and bake for 40 minutes or until the croustade is golden and bubbling. Let it cool for 15 minutes before serving. Serve the croustade warm or at room temperature.

GALAKTOBOUREKO

Serves 12

- 4 cups sugar, divided
- 1 cup water
- 1 tablespoon fresh lemon juice
- 1 tablespoon plus
- 1 1/2 teaspoons grated lemon zest, divided 10 cups whole milk, at room temperature
- 1 cup plus 2 tablespoons unsalted butter, melted and divided 2 tablespoons vanilla extract
- 7 large eggs, at room temperature
- 1 cup fine semolina
- 1 package phyllo, thawed and at room temperature

Directions

- In a medium pot over medium-high heat, bring 2 cups of sugar, water, lemon juice, and 1 1/2 teaspoons lemon zest to a boil. Reduce the heat to medium-low and cook for 10 minutes. Remove the pot from the heat, let syrup come to room temperature, and set it aside.
- Put the milk, 2 tablespoons of butter, the remaining sugar, and vanilla in a large pot over medium-high heat. Cook the mixture until the milk is scalded and take it off the heat.
- In another bowl, whisk the eggs and semolina. Slowly whisk a ladle of milk into the egg mixture. Add four more ladles of milk, one at a time. Transfer the egg mixture into the milk mixture and place the pot over medium heat. Stir

the mixture until it thickens to a consistency like custard. Add the remaining zest and take off the heat. Place a tea towel over the pan, and cover the pan with a lid to prevent a crust from forming. Set it aside.

- Preheat the oven to 350°F. Remove the phyllo from package and divide the sheets into two equal piles (tops and bottoms). Cover each pile with a damp tea towel so the phyllo doesn't dry out. Brush the bottom and sides of a 13" × 9" baking pan with butter.

- Take one sheet of phyllo from the bottom pile, and brush with butter. Place the phyllo sheet in the bottom of the pan with a quarter of the sheet hanging over the sides. Continue buttering and laying the bottom-layer sheets in the pan until the entire bottom and edges are covered with phyllo. Add the custard, spread it evenly over the bottom sheets, then wrap the overhanging phyllo over the custard.

- Take one sheet from the top pile and brush the surface with butter. Place the sheet on top of the filling and repeat the process with the remaining sheets to cover the entire surface of the pan. If excess phyllo is hanging from the edges of the pan, tuck the excess into the sides of the pan. Score the top layers of the phyllo, about 1⁄4-inch deep, into serving squares.

- Bake the pie on the middle rack of the oven for 35–40 minutes or until the top is golden. As soon as the pie is removed from the oven, ladle the reserved syrup over the entire surface. Use all the syrup. Let the galaktoboureko absorb the syrup as it comes to room temperature. Cut it and serve it at room temperature or cold.

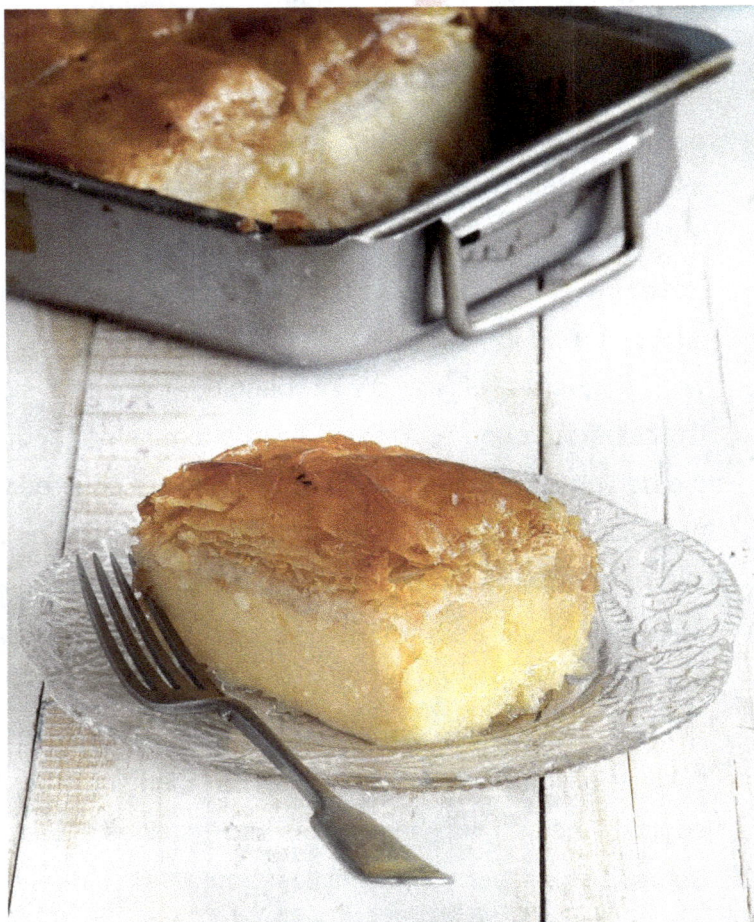

MEDITERRANEAN BREAD

LAHMACUN

Serves 8

- 1/2 large green bell pepper, stemmed, seeded, and chopped 1 medium red onion, peeled and chopped
- 2 cloves garlic, peeled and smashed
- 1 tablespoon red pepper paste
- 1 medium tomato, blanched, peeled, and chopped
- 1/2 pound ground lamb or beef
- 1 teaspoon salt
- 1/2 teaspoon pepper 1/2 teaspoon red pepper flakes
- 1 teaspoon ground allspice
- 1 teaspoon dried oregano
- 1/4 cup extra-virgin olive oil Pizza Dough
- 1/4 cup all-purpose flour

Directions

- Preheat the oven to 450°F. Set a pizza stone on the middle rack to preheat as well. If you don't have a pizza stone, use a large greased baking sheet.
- In a food processor, combine the peppers, onion, garlic, red pepper paste, and tomato. Pulse until the ingredients form a coarse paste. Add the ground lamb or beef, salt, pepper, red pepper flakes, allspice, oregano, and oil.
- Make sure the Pizza Dough has risen in a warm place for 1 1/2–2 hours. Punch down the dough and divide it into three pieces. Work with one piece of dough at a time. While one is baking, assemble the next one. Stretch and

flatten the dough into a long oval shape (about 10" × 4"). Transfer the dough to a well-floured pizza peel (paddle), which is a traditional Italian tool like a wide flat shovel, for moving a pizza so that the dough doesn't stick when you transfer it to the pizza stone (or baking sheet).

- Spread a third of the lamb filling over the top of the dough. Using your fingers, massage the filling into the dough, getting as near to the edges as possible. Carefully slide the lahmacun onto the pizza stone and bake it for 7–8 minutes or until the crust is browned. Repeat with the remaining dough and filling.
- Serve this dish hot or at room temperature.

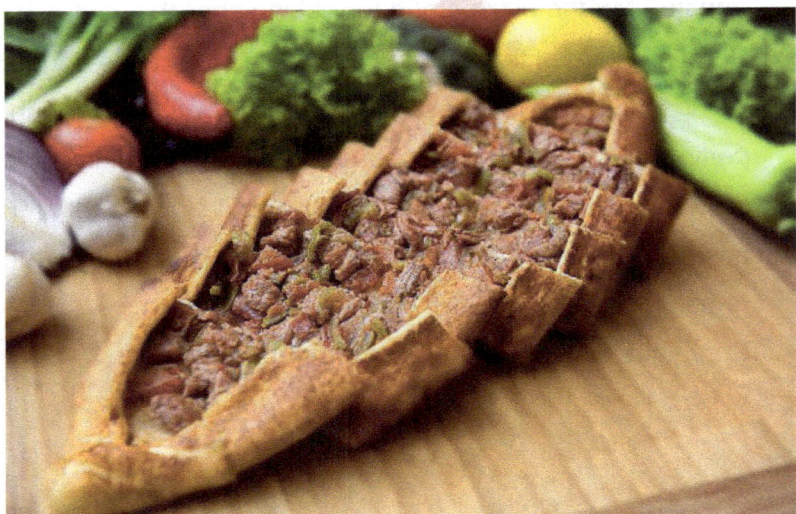

EASY HOMEMADE BREAD

Makes 3 loaves

- 2 tablespoons active dry yeast
- 1 teaspoon sugar
- 3 1/2 cups tepid water
- 6 3/4 cups plus
- 2 tablespoons unbleached all-purpose flour, divided
- 1 1/2 tablespoons salt
- 2 tablespoons coarse semolina flour

Directions

- In a large bowl, combine yeast, sugar, and water. Set aside for 7–10 minutes. Gradually stir in 6 1/2 cups flour and salt until a dough starts to form. If the mixture seems a little dry, add up to 1/2 cup tepid water until the dough comes together. It should feel smooth and not too sticky. Cover the bowl with plastic wrap, leaving a small opening to allow the gases to escape. Let the dough rise a minimum of 2 hours or overnight.
- Sprinkle 1/4 cup flour on a work surface. Divide dough into three pieces and work with one at a time. Stretch the dough outward and then fold under. Repeat this for 2–3 minutes. You should end up with a smooth, round ball (boule) of dough. Repeat with remaining dough.
- Sprinkle the semolina flour over a piece of parchment paper the same size as a pizza stone or baking sheet. Place the boules on the parchment, leaving room in

between to allow the dough to rise. Sprinkle remaining flour over the boules. Let rise for 45 minutes. Use a sharp knife to cut three shallow slices into the top of each boule.

- Preheat the oven to 500°F. Set a pizza stone or large baking sheet on the middle rack to preheat. Add hot water to a broiler pan and place it on the top rack. Transfer the boules to the pizza stone or baking sheet and bake for 5 minutes. Reduce the temperature to 450°F and bake for 20 minutes or until the boules are golden.

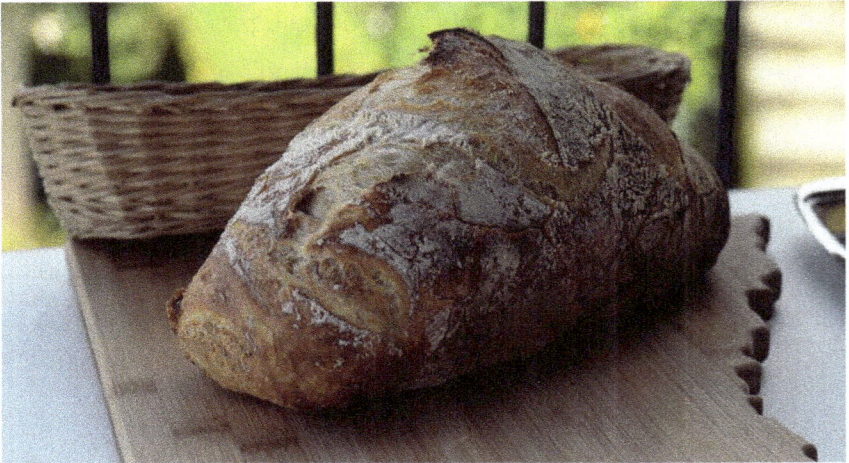

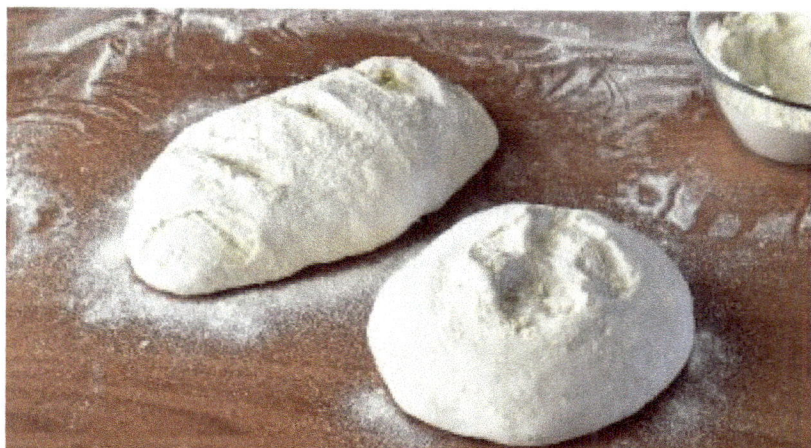

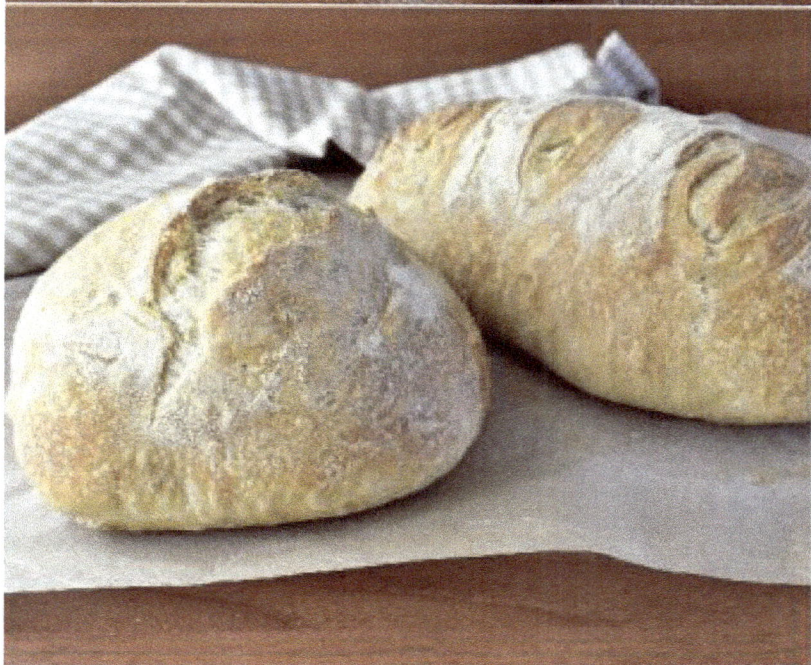

MEDITERRANEAN RICE AND GRAINS

Creamy Corn, Squash and Cilantro

Serves: 8

Ingredients

- 4 cloves garlic, minced and divided
- 1⁄4 cup cilantro, minced
- 1⁄2 cup mayonnaise
- 2 tablespoons sour cream
- 1⁄4 teaspoon salt
- 1 bag (10 oz.) Simple Truth Organic Whole Kernel Cut Corn
- 3 tablespoons Olive oil
- 1 zucchini, washed and chopped
- 1 yellow squash, washed and chopped
- 1⁄2 cup queso fresco, crumbled

Directions

- Heat grill to 250°F.
- To make aioli, mix 2 garlic cloves, mayonnaise, sour cream and salt in a small bowl.
- Cook corn in microwave as directed on the package.
- Heat oil in cast iron skillet and place on the grill. Add 2 minced garlic cloves and cook, uncovered, for 30 seconds. Add zucchini and yellow squash and cook for 3-5 minutes, turning occasionally, until vegetables are crisp-tender. Add corn and cook until vegetables are cooked through.
- Serve vegetables with aioli and queso fresco on the side.

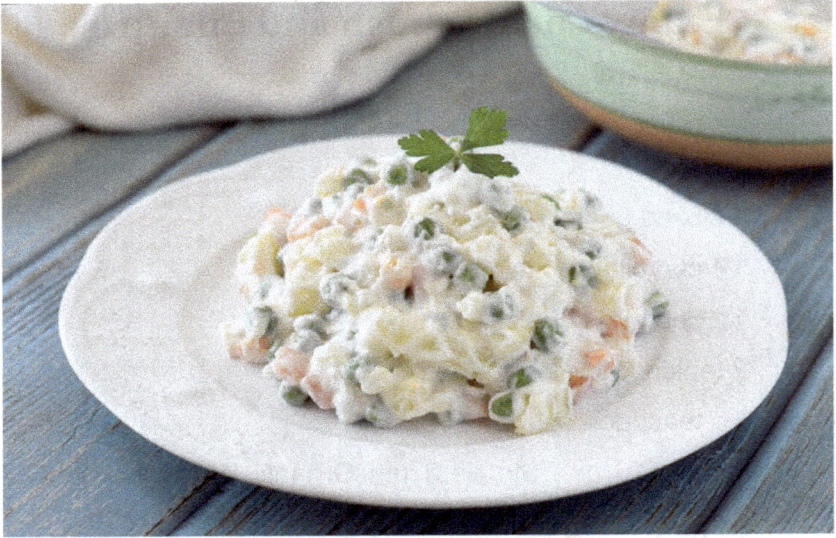

MEDITERRANEAN EGG AND RECIPIES

Mediterranean Egg Mug

Ingredients:

- One farm fresh egg
- 1 Tbsp Trader Joe's Fat Free crumbled Feta cheese (if you don't like Feta sub the Laughing Cow Light Swiss wedge like in my other recipes)
- Diced Mushrooms (I prefer baby bellas)
- Banana pepper rings
- 3 large olives (I try to use Kalamata but black or green work well too)
- Fresh kale and/or baby spinach
- Fresh ground black pepper
- Olive oil non stick spray

Directions

- Spray mug, muffin cooker or crock bowl with non stick spray. Add everything but the egg and cook in microwave on high for 30 seconds
- Crack open egg and add to bowl stirring gently but evenly into the other ingredients.
- Return to microwave for 2 minutes on high. If you have a low wattage microwave or the mixture is still "loose" continue to microwave in 20 second increments until everything is firm but not hard. Add fresh black pepper. Let sit for one minute before trying to remove from bowl to move to bread or plate. The egg "muffin" should slide out

easily.   Use your imagination, these are a delicious and quick filling breakfast…enjoy!

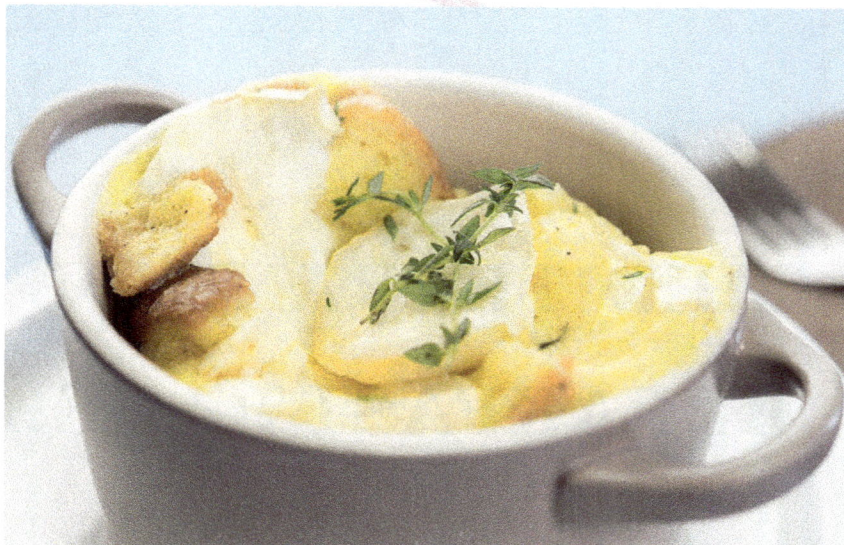

MEDITERRANEAN BREAKFAST BAKE

Keto Garlic Cheese Bread Recipe

An easy keto cheese bread recipe with gooey cheese pulls! Low carb keto garlic cheese bread with almond flour or coconut flour tastes like the real thing, but has only 3g net carbs.

Ingredients

Fathead dough:

- 3 cups Mozzarella cheese (shredded)
- 2 oz Cream cheese (cut into cubes)
- 1 1/2 cupsWholesome Yum Blanched Almond Flour
- 2 large Eggs
- 1/2 tbspGluten-free baking powder

Optional yeast ingredients:

- 1 packetActive dry yeast (2 1/4 tsp)
- 1/4 cup Water (lukewarm)
- 1 tspInulin powder

Topping:

- 2 tbspButter (melted)
- 1/2 tspItalian seasoning
- 1/2 tspGarlic powder
- 1 1/2 cups Mozzarella cheese (shredded)

Instructions

1. Preheat the oven to 350 degrees F (176 degrees C). Line a baking sheet with parchment paper.

2. If you want to include the optional yeast, stir the warm water, inulin, and yeast in a small bowl, and set aside for 10-15 minutes to bloom.

3. Meanwhile, process the almond flour, baking powder, and eggs in a food processor.

4. Melt the mozzarella and cream cheese together in a bowl in the microwave (90 seconds, stirring halfway through and at the end) or a double boiler on the stove (stirring occasionally until smooth).

5. Immediately before the cheeses cool, add them to the food processor with the blade placed over the cheese, and process until a dough forms.

6. Once the yeast looks frothy and puffy, add it to the food processor. Pulse until just combined.

7. If the dough feels sticky to the touch, chill it for 15-30 minutes, until it feels firmer and less sticky.

8. Using oiled hands to make the dough easier to work with, form a ball and then flatten into a disc (3/4 inch tall, 7 inch diameter) on the parchment lined baking sheet. If the dough is sticky again after forming the disc, you may need to chill it again so that it's less sticky.

9. Use a knife to cut rows one inch apart in the dough disc, cutting almost to the bottom but not all the way through. Then, cut 1 inch apart in the perpendicular direction, to form a grid, again not cutting all the way through.

10. In a small bowl, stir together the melted butter, Italian seasoning, and garlic powder. Brush over the dough, letting it drip down into the cuts you made. Stuff shredded

mozzarella inside the cuts, trying to avoid a 1/2 inch border at the edges, so that it doesn't seep out during baking (it's okay if a little gets in).

11. Bake for 15-18 minutes, until the cheesy bread is golden and cooked through.

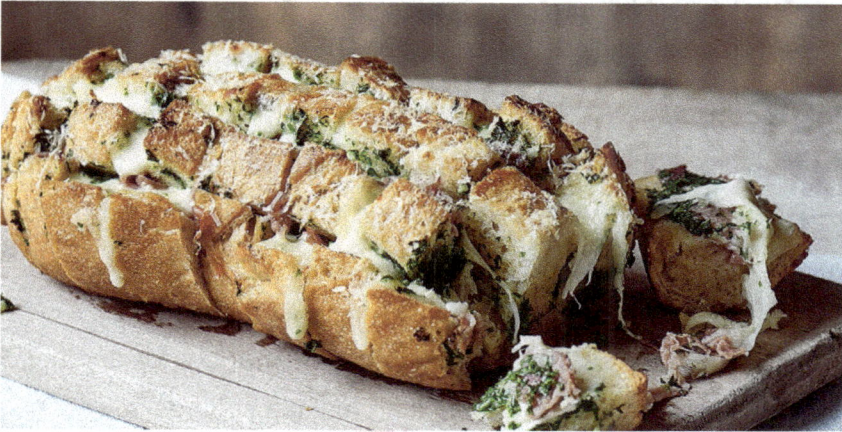

Keto Cloud Bread - Low Carb Burger Buns

Ingredients

- 4 Large Eggs
- 1/2 tsp Cream Of Tartar
- 1/4 Cup Cream Cheese
- 1/2 tsp Salt
- 1/2 tsp Garlic Powder (Optional)

Instructions

1. Crack the eggs and seperate the whites from the yolks. Put all the whites into a bowl and whisk with an electric mixer for 1 - 2 mins.
2. egg whites in a bowl
3. Add the Cream Of Tartar and whisk again for another 1 min. The mixture should start making soft peaks
4. cream of tatar with egg whites
5. In another bowl, add the yolks, salt, cream cheese and garlic powder (optional), mixing on high until well combined. Gently fold this mixture into the egg whites.
6. combine egg yolks into egg whites
7. Spoon out the final mixture onto a tray lined with baking paper. They do fluff up a bit in the oven so leave enough space to breathe!
8. cloud bread tray
9. Put in the oven at 180 c (375F) for 15-20 mins until slightly golden brown on top. Serve and enjoy!

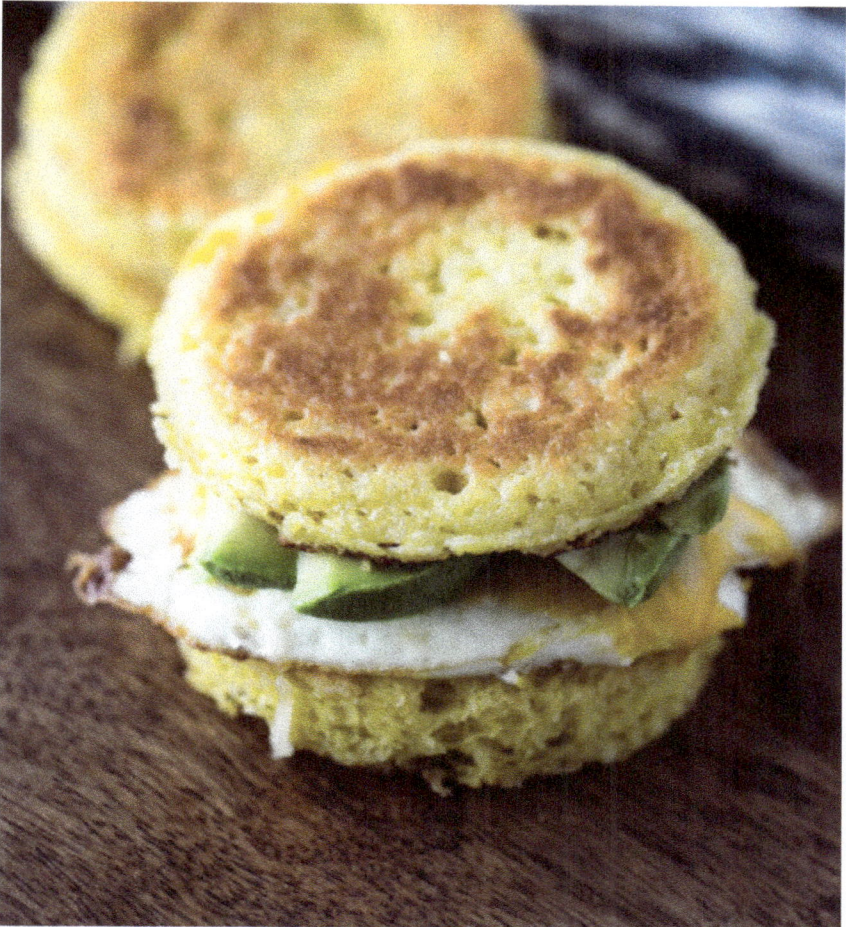

Keto Coconut Bread

Ingredients

- 7 Large Eggs
- 1/2 cup Coconut Flour
- 1/2 cup Butter 120g / 4 oz (use 1/2 cup olive/coconut oil for dairy free)
- 1/4 tsp Salt
- 1/4 tsp baking powder (aluminium free if possible)
- 1/2 tsp xanthan gum (optional)

Instructions

1. Preheat oven to 180 C (355 F).
2. Crack the eggs into a bowl and mix for 1 minute until well combined.
3. Add the coconut flour, butter, salt, baking powder and xanthan gum, and mix until completely combined. The mixture will become quite thick.
4. Line an 8.5 X 5-inch (21.5 x 12.7 cm) loaf tin with parchment paper and pour the batter into the tin. Level the top with a spatula if uneven.
5. Bake for 50 minutes or until a skewer comes out of the middle clean.
6. Nutrition information is for 1 slice. Slice and store in the fridge for up to 5 days or in the freezer for up to 2 weeks. This bread freezes well.

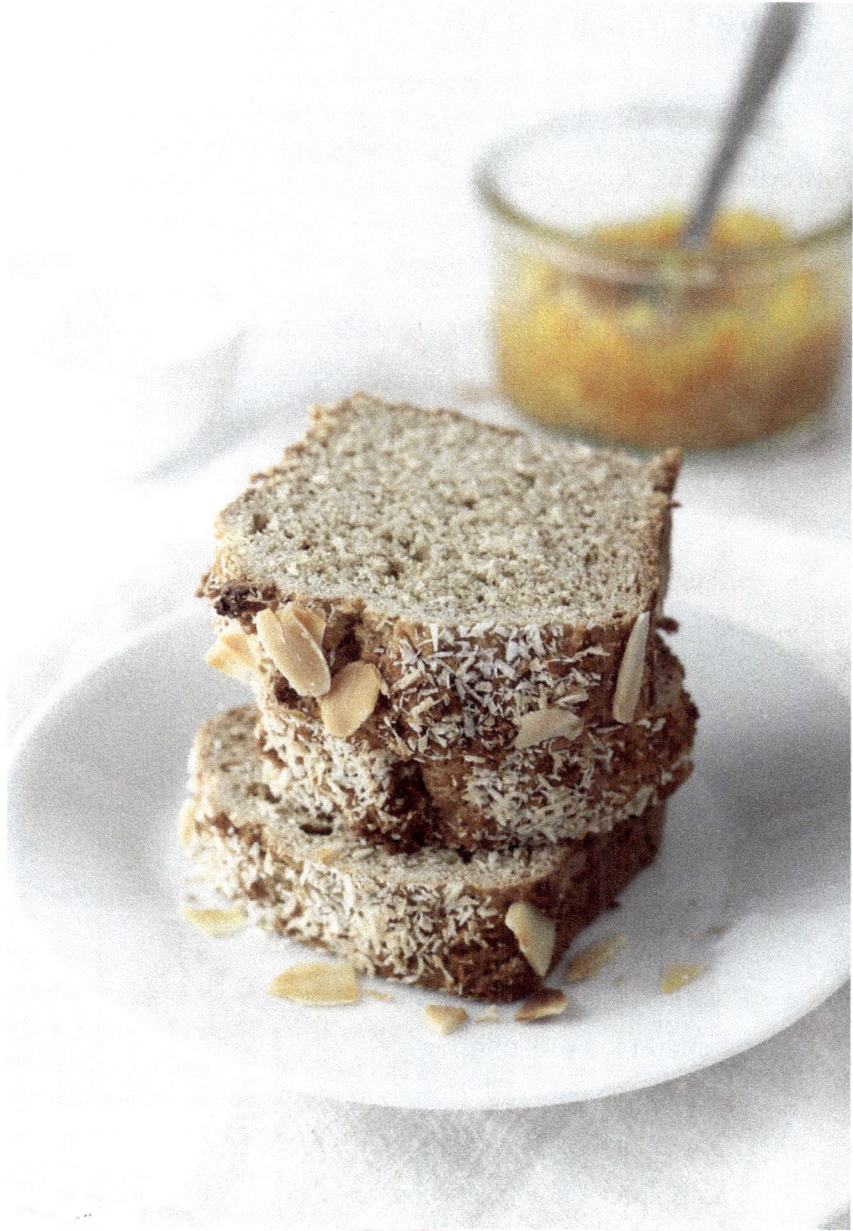

Low Carb Bread Recipe - Keto Seeded Bread

Ingredients

- 7 large Eggs
- 2 Cups Almond Flour 170g / 6 oz
- 1/2 Cup unsalted butter 100g / 3.5 oz
- 2 Tbsp olive oil 30ml / 1 fl oz
- 2 Tbsp Chia Seeds
- 3 Tbsp Sesame Seeds
- 1 tsp baking powder
- 1/2 tsp xanthan gum
- 1/4 tsp Salt

Instructions

1. Preheat oven to 180C (355F)
2. In a medium mixing bowl, whisk the large eggs together.
3. Add the remaining ingredients, and mix together well. Using an electric hand whisk often helps with this recipe as the mixture can become quite thick.
4. Pour into a loaf tin lined with baking paper. Place sesame seeds on top (optional)
5. Bake for 40 minutes. (Remove once a skewer comes out of the middle clean).
6. Can be sliced into 16 slices. Best kept in the fridge for up to 5 days, or frozen for up to 3 weeks.

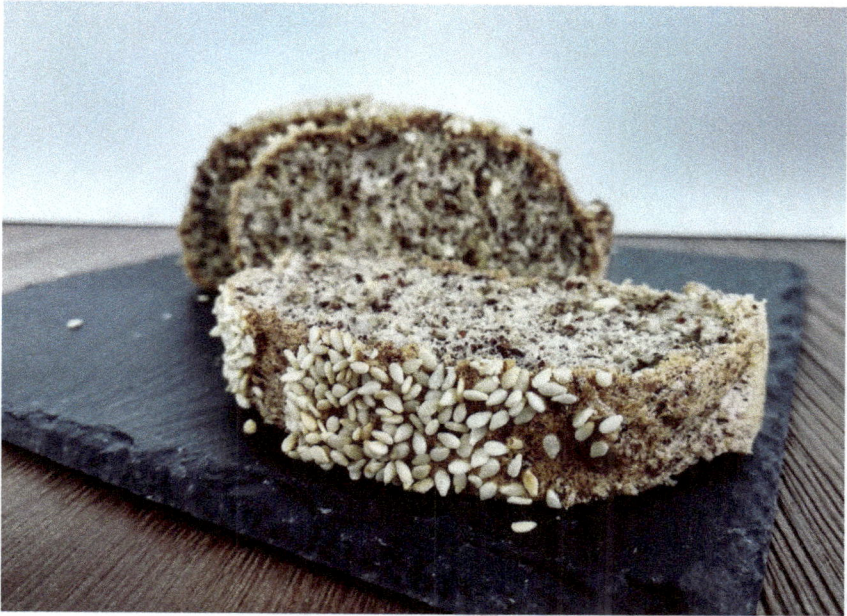

MEDITERRANEAN APPETIZERS

Healthy Nachos

Total time: 12 minutes

Prep time: 10 minutes

Cook time: 2 minutes

Yields: 6 servings

Ingredients

- 1 medium green onion, thinly sliced (about 1 tbsp.)
- 1 finely chopped and drained plum tomato
- 2 tsp. oil from container of sun-dried tomatoes
- 2 tbsp. sun-dried tomatoes in oil, finely chopped
- 2 tbsp. Kalamata olives, finely chopped
- 4 oz. restaurant-style corn tortilla chips
- 1 (4-oz) package finely crumbled feta cheese

Directions

- Mix together onion, plum tomato, oil, sun-dried tomatoes and olives in a small bowl; set aside.
- Arrange the tortillas chips on a microwavable plate in a single layer; evenly top with cheese and microwave on high for 1 minute.
- Rotate the plate half turn and continue microwaving for 30 more seconds or until cheese is bubbly.
- Evenly spread the tomato mixture over the chips and cheese and serve.

Jalapeno Boats

Total time: 35 minutes

Prep time: 10 minutes

Cook time: 25 minutes

Yields: 44 servings

Ingredients

- 1 bag (12 oz.) vegetarian burger crumbles
- 1 cup Parmesan cheese, shredded
- 1 package (8 oz.) softened light cream cheese
- 22 large jalapeno peppers, cut into halves lengthwise and seeds removed

Directions

- Sauté crumbles in a large skillet set over medium heat for about 5 minutes or until heated through.
- Combine together shredded Parmesan and softened cream cheese in a small bowl; fold in the crumble.
- Preheat oven to 425°F. Spoon about 1 tablespoon of the crumble-cheese mixture into each jalapeno half; arrange the jalapeno halves on a baking sheet, cheese side up, and bake in preheated oven for about 20 minutes or until the filling is bubbly and lightly browned.